© [DEHART HAIRSTON], [2024]

All rights reserved. No part of this publication may be reproduced, distributed, or transmitted in any form or by any means, including photocopying, recording, or other electronic or mechanical methods, without the prior written permission of the publisher, except in the case of brief quotations embodied in critical reviews and certain other noncommercial uses permitted by copyright law.

DISCLAIMER

This book's content is only intended for general informative purposes. At the time of writing, the author has taken every precaution to guarantee that the material is correct and current. Nevertheless, the author disclaims all explicit and implicit representations and guarantees about the availability, appropriateness, correctness, completeness, and usefulness of the material on these pages.

Since the author is not a licensed medical practitioner, the material in this book shouldn't be interpreted as medical advice. Before making any modifications to their diet, exercise regimen, or medical treatment, readers are urged to speak with a licensed healthcare provider.

Moreover, the author has no connection to any of the businesses, organizations, or people that are discussed in this book. Any mentions of goods, services, businesses, or people are purely informative and do not indicate endorsement or suggestion.

This book's content is entirely dependent on the author's expertise, study, and comprehension of the topic. Despite having taken reasonable care to offer correct information, the author disclaims all liability for any mistakes or omissions in the material as well as for any losses, harm, or damages resulting from using the information.

It is recommended that readers use their own judgment and discretion when applying the knowledge in this book to their own situations. The use or implementation of any material in this book may result in unfavorable repercussions, directly or indirectly, for which the author assumes no liability.

By reading this book, you agree to release and hold the author harmless from any claims, losses, liabilities, costs, or expenditures resulting from or related to the use of the information you get from it.

Table of Contents

CHAPTER 1 13
- Understanding Digestion 13
- Introduction To The Digestive System 13
- Function Of The Stomach 14
- Importance Of Gastric Acid 15
- Overview Of Peptic Ulcers 16

CHAPTER 2 19
- Causes And Risk Factors 19
- H. Pylori Infection 19
- Nonsteroidal Anti-Inflammatory Drugs (Nsaids) ..20
- Stress And Lifestyle Factors 21
- Genetic Predisposition 23

CHAPTER 3 25
- Signs And Symptoms 25
- Burning Pain In The Stomach 25
- Stomach Pain That Burns 25
- Feeling Queasy And Throwing Up 26
- Burping And Bloating 26
- Stools That Are Black And Bleed 27

CHAPTER 4 29

Diagnosis **29**
Medical History And Physical Examination **29**
Endoscopy And Biopsy **30**
Imaging Tests (X-Ray, Ct Scan) **31**
Laboratory Tests (H. Pylori Detection) **32**

CHAPTER 5 .... **35**
Treatment Options **35**
Medications (Proton Pump Inhibitors, Antibiotics)
.... **35**
Lifestyle Changes (Diet, Stress Management) **36**
Surgical Intervention (Rare Cases) **37**
Alternative Therapies (Probiotics, Herbal Remedies) **38**

CHAPTER 6 .... **41**
Complications **41**
Bleeding Ulcers **41**
Perforation **42**
Obstruction **44**
Increased Risk Of Stomach Cancer **45**

CHAPTER 7 .... **49**
Prevention Strategies **49**
H. Pylori Eradication **49**

Reducing The Use Of Nsaids 51
Healthy Diet And Lifestyle Habits 53
Regular Screening For High-Risk Individuals 55
CHAPTER 8 57
Diet And Nutrition 57
Foods To Avoid (Spicy, Acidic) 57
Foods To Consume (Fiber-Rich, Probiotics) 58
Meal Planning Tips For Ulcer Management 60
   1. Balanced Plate: 60
   2. Small, Frequent Meals: 60
   3. Mindful Eating: 61
   4. Reduce Food Triggers: 61
   5. Keep Yourself Hydrated: 61
Hydration Importance 62
CHAPTER 9 65
Coping And Support 65
Psychological Impact Of Peptic Ulcers 65
Stress Management Techniques 66
Communicating With Healthcare Providers 68
CHAPTER 10 71
Living With Peptic Ulcers 71

Long-Term Outlook 71
Monitoring For Recurrence 73
Quality Of Life Considerations 75
Resources For Ongoing Education And Support ... 77
CONCLUSION 80
THE END 83

ABOUT THE BOOK

"Peptic Ulcers" is more than simply a book; it's a vital resource that clarifies a problem that affects millions of people globally. This book covers all the bases, from the fundamentals of digestion to managing the day-to-day difficulties of having peptic ulcers.

The complex functions of the digestive system are explained to readers in Chapter 1, which also highlights the critical function of stomach acid and how an imbalance in it may result in peptic ulcers. Comprehending this basis is essential to understanding the next chapters.

In Chapter 2, the causes and risk factors—which range from H. pylori infection to genetic predispositions and lifestyle decisions. Equipped with this understanding, perusers may recognize plausible catalysts and proactively address hazards.

Understanding the symptoms and indicators, as described in Chapter 3, is essential to obtaining prompt medical attention. Knowing these signals, which range from the traditional burning pain to concerning indicators like bleeding, might help avoid consequences.

To make an accurate diagnosis, Chapter 4 walks readers through the diagnostic procedure and emphasizes the use of a complete medical history, and exact testing like endoscopy, and biopsy.

The Chapter 5 treatment alternatives provide comfort and hope. Readers are provided with a wide range of techniques that are customized to meet their specific requirements, ranging from medicine to lifestyle modifications.

Readers may travel with care and awareness if they are aware of the possible issues, as explained in Chapter 6.

Preventive techniques, discussed in Chapter 7, are equally important since they emphasize the need to take proactive steps to stop peptic ulcers from developing or returning.

Chapter 8 on food and nutrition offers helpful advice on how to maintain a stomach-friendly diet and improve general health.

Providing important insights into coping strategies, networks of support, and long-term care, Chapters 9 and 10 highlight the complete approach required to live effectively with peptic ulcers.

"Peptic Ulcers" is a lifeline for anyone navigating the complexity of this ailment, not simply a book. Regardless of your role in healthcare—as a patient, caregiver, or professional—its thorough coverage and useful guidance make it an invaluable tool on your path to recovery and well-being.

CHAPTER 1

Understanding Digestion

Introduction To The Digestive System

The job of the digestive system, a marvelously intricate network of organs and tissues, is to convert food into nutrients that the body can absorb and use for growth, repair, and energy. It is made up of many associated organs that are essential to the process of digestion, such as the liver, gallbladder, pancreas, stomach, esophagus, small and large intestines, mouth, and gallbladder.

The stomach, a muscular organ in the upper left area of the belly, is the central component of this system. Food is stored in the stomach, where it is combined with gastric secretions and churned into a semi-liquid material called chyme. Subsequently, the combination is progressively discharged into the small intestine to facilitate further digestion and absorption.

Function Of The Stomach

The stomach performs several crucial tasks during digestion. First of all, it serves as a place to store food, enabling us to eat bigger meals than our bodies could quickly digest. Second, it secretes gastric secretions that aid in the breakdown of food into smaller pieces that are easier to absorb. These fluids include hydrochloric acid and enzymes. Furthermore, the stomach's acidic environment helps to sterilize food by destroying potentially dangerous microorganisms.

As food passes through the digestive system more easily and is combined with gastric fluids, the muscular walls of the stomach flex regularly. The term "peristalsis" refers to this mechanism that aids in ensuring complete food particle mixing and digestion.

Importance Of Gastric Acid

Hydrochloric acid (HCl), a vital component of gastric juice, is essential to the process of digestion. Among its many uses are the activation of digestive enzymes, the conversion of proteins into amino acids, and the elimination of potential foodborne microorganisms.

Digestive enzymes like pepsin, which must have an acidic pH to be active, work best in an acidic environment, which is provided by the stomach. Inadequate stomach acid production may hinder digestion and cause insufficient absorption of nutrients.

On the other hand, overproduction of stomach acid may also be harmful, perhaps resulting in peptic ulcers or gastroesophageal reflux disease (GERD).

For the health of the digestive system, the generation of stomach acid must be balanced.

Overview Of Peptic Ulcers

Peptic ulcers are lesions that form on the esophageal, small intestine, or stomach lining due to acid reflux from the stomach. The symptoms of these ulcers might include heartburn, nausea, vomiting, bloating, and stomach discomfort. They can also vary in size and intensity.

Helicobacter pylori (H. pylori) infection or chronic use of nonsteroidal anti-inflammatory medicines (NSAIDs) like aspirin or ibuprofen are thought to be the main causes of peptic ulcers. Ulcers may also occur as a result of other causes including stress, smoking, and binge drinking.

If left untreated, peptic ulcers may result in bleeding, intestinal or stomach perforation, and in rare instances, stomach cancer.

Therefore, to obtain the right care and avoid further difficulties, it is imperative that you consult a doctor if you feel any of the symptoms of a peptic ulcer.

Maintaining digestive health and avoiding digestive problems need an understanding of the processes involved in digestion, the formation of gastric acid, and the development of peptic ulcers. A balanced diet, frequent exercise, and stress-reduction methods are all important components of a healthy lifestyle that may promote good digestive function and lower the chance of developing peptic ulcers.

CHAPTER 2

Causes And Risk Factors

H. Pylori Infection

H. The bacterium known as Helicobacter pylori, or pylori, affects the lining of the stomach. It is among the most typical reasons why peptic ulcers occur. This bacterium is often picked up in infancy, most frequently via tainted food or drink, and if untreated, it may linger for many years.

The fact that H is present. gastrointestinal pylori may cause inflammation and harm to the stomach's protective lining, increasing the stomach's vulnerability to the corrosive effects of stomach acid. Peptic ulcers may ultimately develop as a consequence of this. Even However, not everyone has an H infection. Pylori will result in ulcers; this risk is greatly increased by the bacterium.

Making the diagnosis H. An endoscopy, blood test, stool test, or breath test are usually used to diagnose pylori infection. Antibiotics and acid-suppressing drugs are often used in conjunction with treatment to get rid of the bacteria and encourage ulcer repair.

Nonsteroidal Anti-Inflammatory Drugs (Nsaids)

NSAIDs, or nonsteroidal anti-inflammatory medicines, are often used to treat inflammation and alleviate pain. NSAIDs work well for a variety of ailments, but long-term usage or excessive dosages may raise the risk of peptic ulcers.

NSAIDs function by preventing the cyclooxygenases (COX) enzymes from producing prostaglandins, which are compounds that help protect the stomach lining.

Because NSAIDs inhibit prostaglandin synthesis, they may increase the stomach's susceptibility to acid reflux disease.

Peptic ulcers are more common in those who routinely use NSAIDs, such as aspirin, ibuprofen, or naproxen, particularly in large amounts or over extended periods. Older persons and those with a history of stomach bleeding or ulcers are at an even higher risk.

Doctors could advise taking the lowest effective dosage for the shortest amount of time required to lower the risk of NSAID-induced ulcers. Furthermore, for those who are very susceptible, it can be advisable to transfer to a new class of drugs or use alternate pain management techniques.

Stress And Lifestyle Factors

Although lifestyle choices and stress may not directly cause peptic ulcers, they can worsen symptoms and aid in their development. Prolonged stress, unhealthy eating habits, smoking, excessive alcohol intake, and irregular meal schedules may all negatively impact the gastrointestinal tract's health and make ulcers more likely.

Stress, either mental or physical, may alter the motility and production of stomach acid, which can exacerbate pre-existing ulcers or cause symptoms in those who are vulnerable. Furthermore, bad lifestyle choices like smoking and binge drinking may erode the stomach lining's protective layer against acid erosion.

Peptic ulcer risk may be decreased and overall gastrointestinal health can be improved by leading a healthy lifestyle that includes regular exercise, a balanced diet, stress management practices, abstaining from smoking and excessive alcohol use, and stress management strategies.

Genetic Predisposition

A person's vulnerability to peptic ulcers may also be influenced by genetic factors. Genes may affect the thickness of the stomach lining, the development of protective mucus, and the sensitivity to H, but not everyone with a family history of ulcers will develop them. NSAID usage or H. pylori infection.

Individuals may be more susceptible to increased inflammatory responses or compromised healing processes as a result of certain genetic variants, which might increase their chance of developing ulcers in response to environmental stimuli. Comprehending an individual's genetic susceptibility to ulcers may facilitate the development of tailored treatment plans and preventative strategies.

It's important to keep in mind, too, that lifestyle choices and environmental variables are just as important in the development of peptic ulcers as heredity is. People may lower their chances of getting ulcers and preserve good gastrointestinal health by proactively addressing both inherited predispositions and modifiable risk factors.

CHAPTER 3

Signs And Symptoms

Burning Pain In The Stomach

Even though they are often accompanied by pain and discomfort, peptic ulcers may present with a wide range of signs and symptoms, thus early detection is essential for effective management and treatment. Recognizing possible ulcers and getting the right medical care may be greatly aided by being aware of these symptoms.

Stomach Pain That Burns

Constant burning in the stomach region is one of the main signs of peptic ulcers. Most people describe this discomfort as a slow, gnawing aching that may become worse or go away over time. It usually happens when the stomach is empty, either throughout the night or in between meals.

An individual's quality of life may be greatly affected by this burning feeling, which can be felt anywhere from the navel to the breastbone and continue for minutes to many hours.

Feeling Queasy And Throwing Up

Those who have peptic ulcers often feel nausea and vomiting as symptoms. The ulcer's irritation and inflammation might make you feel sick to your stomach and want to throw up. Vomiting may sometimes provide momentary respite from the pain brought on by the ulcer. Nonetheless, prolonged nausea and vomiting should be evaluated medically to rule out complications or underlying diseases, particularly if they are accompanied by other symptoms.

Burping And Bloating

Additionally, bloating and frequent burping may result from peptic ulcers. Bloating and gas accumulation may result from regular digestion being disrupted by the ulcer and increased production of stomach acid. The body may try to release extra gas by burping often along with this bloating feeling. While occasional burping and bloating are typical body processes, persistent or severe symptoms call for a visit to the doctor to rule out any underlying conditions like peptic ulcers.

Stools That Are Black And Bleed

Blood may be seen in stools or vomit in more severe instances of peptic ulcers due to hemorrhage. Melena, or black, tarry stools, are a common side effect of bleeding ulcers that show that there is blood in the gastrointestinal system that has been digested. Since this symptom might indicate severe bleeding and possible problems including anemia or hemorrhage, it needs to be treated immediately.

To address the underlying cause of bleeding and stop further problems, prompt examination and treatment are crucial.

It is essential to comprehend and identify the symptoms and indicators linked to peptic ulcers to seek prompt medical attention and treatment. Even though each person may experience these symptoms differently and to varying degrees, early identification and treatment may help reduce pain, encourage healing, and avert problems related to peptic ulcers. If you have any of these symptoms or are worried about the health of your digestive system, get in touch with a medical practitioner for an appropriate assessment and needs-specific advice.

CHAPTER 4

Diagnosis

Medical History And Physical Examination

Your road toward a diagnosis of peptic ulcers usually starts with a comprehensive medical history and physical examination. Your symptoms, their length, and any circumstances that can aggravate or lessen them will be important information for your doctor to know. The setting up of further diagnostic procedures and treatment strategies is what makes this talk so important.

Your doctor would probably concentrate on your abdomen area while doing the physical examination. To feel discomfort or sensitivity that would point to the existence of an ulcer, they can lightly push several locations. They could also ask about other symptoms, such as nausea, bloating, or weight loss, which might give important hints about your health.

Endoscopy And Biopsy

An essential diagnostic technique for peptic ulcers is endoscopy. An endoscope, which is a thin, flexible tube with a camera at the tip, is put into your mouth and used to guide the tube down your neck, into your stomach, duodenum, and esophagus. This enables your physician to visually assess these organs for anomalies, such as ulcers.

Your doctor could take a biopsy if an ulcer is found during the endoscopy. To do this, a little sample of tissue from the ulcerated region must be taken for further microscopic inspection. Biopsies are necessary to rule out other illnesses, such as stomach cancer, and to confirm the diagnosis of peptic ulcers.

Imaging Tests (X-Ray, Ct Scan)

Your doctor could sometimes prescribe imaging studies to help with the peptic ulcer diagnosis. Your gastrointestinal system may be seen in great detail on X-rays and CT scans, which can assist detect ulcers and determine their size and location. These imaging examinations are especially helpful when endoscopy is not possible or cannot provide sufficient results.

You will be asked to lie on a table while X-ray pictures are obtained for an abdominal X-ray. Certain signs, such as air- or fluid-filled cavities in the stomach or duodenum, that are indicative of ulcers may be shown by this non-invasive method. By combining X-rays from various angles, CT scans provide even more comprehensive pictures and a three-dimensional perspective of your digestive system.

Laboratory Tests (H. Pylori Detection)

H. Peptic ulcers are often caused by Helicobacter pylori infections. As a result, identifying the existence of these bacteria is essential for a precise diagnosis and the right course of action. To detect H, laboratory testing is essential. pylori throughout your body.

One typical test for H. The urea breath test is called pylori. You will be given a special drink to drink during the test that contains a safe type of radioactive carbon. Should H. If you have H. pylori in your stomach, it will break down the urea in the drink and release carbon dioxide, which is what you smell like.

An additional approach for H. A stool antigen test is used to identify pylori. This entails supplying a stool sample, which is then examined to see if H is present. antigens of pylori.

If the bacteria is there, certain H-related proteins. You will be able to identify pylori in your feces.

Antibodies against H may also be found by blood testing. pylori inside your blood. It is noteworthy, however, that these antibodies may persist even after the illness has been well treated, making blood testing an unreliable means of assessing the efficacy of therapy.

CHAPTER 5

Treatment Options

Medications (Proton Pump Inhibitors, Antibiotics)

One of the most important treatments for peptic ulcers is the use of proton pump inhibitors or PPIs. These medications function by preventing the stomach's acid-producing enzyme system from functioning, which lowers stomach acidity and promotes ulcer healing. Omeprazole, lansoprazole, and esomeprazole are three PPIs that are often given. These drugs are very good at encouraging ulcer healing and preventing recurrence. They are often given once a day, generally before breakfast.

Since Helicobacter pylori (H. pylori) is a prominent cause of peptic ulcers, antibiotics are often recommended in addition to PPIs in instances of H. pylori infection.

PPIs are used in conjunction with antibiotics including metronidazole, amoxicillin, and clarithromycin to remove the H. pylori germs and stop the recurrence of ulcers. Known as triple treatment, this combo therapy is usually administered for a period of one to two weeks.

It's crucial to follow your doctor's instructions precisely while taking medicine and to finish the whole course of therapy, even if your symptoms get better before the recommended dosage is reached. Antibiotic resistance may result from not finishing the whole course of therapy, which would reduce the efficacy of subsequent antibiotic regimens.

Lifestyle Changes (Diet, Stress Management)

Apart from pharmaceuticals, certain lifestyle modifications may aid in the management and avoidance of peptic ulcers. Dietary changes that minimize stomach lining irritation and encourage ulcer healing include avoiding spicy and acidic meals as well as alcohol. Large meals should be avoided in favor of smaller, more frequent meals throughout the day to assist lessen the formation of stomach acid and ease symptoms.

Deep breathing exercises, yoga, and mindfulness meditation are a few stress-reduction strategies that may help lower stress levels, which can worsen the symptoms of peptic ulcers. Incorporating regular physical exercise into your routine and getting enough sleep each night may also help manage stress and improve general health.

Surgical Intervention (Rare Cases)

The majority of peptic ulcers respond well to medication and lifestyle modifications, but in a small number of instances, surgery may be required. Surgery is usually reserved for problems including bleeding, perforation, or blockage of the digestive system, or for ulcers that do not respond to conservative treatment methods.

Procedures like a gastrectomy, which includes removing a portion of the stomach, or a vagotomy, which involves severing the vagus nerve to lessen the generation of acid in the stomach, are surgical alternatives for peptic ulcers. These operations are often only advised as a last resort or when all other therapeutic alternatives have been tried and there is a high risk of consequences.

Alternative Therapies (Probiotics, Herbal Remedies)

Some people may decide to investigate complementary therapies in addition to traditional medical treatments for the treatment of peptic ulcers. Probiotics, which are helpful bacteria that may help restore balance to the gut microbiome, have been shown to benefit some patients with their symptoms, however further study is required to validate the efficacy of these treatments.

Herbal treatments for peptic ulcers may also sometimes be utilized, such as chamomile, aloe vera, and licorice root. Herbal medicines may not be healthy for everyone and may combine with other prescriptions, so it's vital to take care while taking them.

It's crucial to speak with a healthcare professional before beginning any alternative treatment to be sure it's suitable and safe for your particular circumstances. While they may be used in addition to traditional medical care to assist in controlling symptoms and encourage recovery, alternative treatments shouldn't be utilized in place of it.

CHAPTER 6

Complications

Bleeding Ulcers

One of the most worrisome peptic ulcer aftereffects is bleeding. There may be minor to severe bleeding as a result of the ulcer wearing away at the stomach or duodenum's lining. Hematemesis, or vomiting blood, is one symptom of bleeding ulcers. Other symptoms include feeling weak and lightheaded from blood loss and passing black, tarry stools (melena). Due to the potential for life-threatening acute bleeding, this condition needs prompt medical intervention.

Stabilizing the patient's condition is frequently the first step in treating bleeding ulcers, and this may include giving them blood transfusions to recover lost blood volume.

By cauterizing the ulcer or injecting drugs to encourage clotting, endoscopic treatments may also be used to halt the bleeding. Surgery can be required in certain circumstances to close the ulcer and halt the bleeding.

Controlling risk factors, such as avoiding nonsteroidal anti-inflammatory medicines (NSAIDs), giving up smoking, and consuming less alcohol, is essential to preventing bleeding ulcers. Medication may be recommended to patients who have previously had bleeding ulcers to lessen the production of stomach acid and encourage ulcer healing.

Perforation

When an ulcer tears a hole in the stomach or duodenum's wall, it might result in a dangerous consequence known as a perforation. This makes it possible for food and stomach acid to seep into the abdominal cavity, which may result in peritonitis, a serious infection of the lining of the abdomen.

Usually, sudden, intense stomach pain that may spread to the back is the first symptom of a perforated ulcer. Additionally, patients may feel stiffness in their abdomens, as well as an accelerated pulse. A perforation is a medical emergency that has to be repaired and the abdominal cavity cleaned right away by surgery.

Patients with perforated ulcers may be prescribed antibiotics in addition to surgery to prevent or cure peritonitis. To aid in their recuperation, they may also need to get intravenous fluids and pain medication. Patients must see their doctor for follow-up after therapy to track their progress and avoid further issues.

Managing underlying risk factors for peptic ulcers, such as H infection, is necessary to prevent perforation. the H. pylori bacteria or using NSAIDs. Medication that lowers stomach acid production and encourages ulcer healing may be beneficial for patients who are at high risk of perforating.

Obstruction

Peptic ulcers may also result in blockage, particularly if they are situated close to the duodenal entrance or in the stomach's pylorus. Food cannot flow from the stomach into the small intestine due to swelling and scarring from the ulcer. This condition is known as obstruction.

Gastric outlet blockage may cause bloating, nausea, vomiting, and a sense of fullness even after consuming small quantities of food. Inadequate absorption of nutrients may also lead to weight loss and malnourishment in patients. Severe blockage may need hospitalization for fluid replacement due to electrolyte abnormalities and dehydration.

Endoscopic dilation is one possible treatment for gastric outlet blockage, which entails enlarging the restricted region to facilitate easier passage of food. Surgery could be required in some situations to heal the ulcer and remove scar tissue. To maintain appropriate nutrition during their recuperation, patients could also need nutritional assistance, such as feeding tubes or intravenous fluids.

To avoid scar tissue formation and digestive system constriction, prompt treatment of peptic ulcers is necessary to prevent blockage. Dietary adjustments, such as eating smaller, more often meals and avoiding foods that are difficult to digest, may be beneficial for patients who are at risk for blockage.

Increased Risk Of Stomach Cancer

Long-term untreated peptic ulcers may raise the chance of developing stomach cancer, even though the majority of peptic ulcers are benign and heal without problems. Prolonged inflammation brought on by H. Prolonged ulceration or an infection with the pylori bacteria might cause alterations in the stomach lining that eventually could result in cancer.

Individuals who have had peptic ulcers in the past should be routinely screened for stomach cancer, particularly if they have risk factors including a family history of the illness or symptoms that don't go away after treatment. Endoscopy along with biopsy is one screening technique that may be used to check for malignant alterations in the stomach lining.

In those with peptic ulcers, treating underlying risk factors like H is crucial to preventing stomach cancer. Stomach ulcer disease or long-term NSAID usage. Individuals who have a positive H test. Antibiotics may be used to treat pylori to get rid of the bacteria and lower the chance of developing cancer. Furthermore, people with a history of peptic ulcers may benefit from lifestyle changes such as stopping smoking and adhering to a healthy diet, since these may help reduce the risk of stomach cancer.

CHAPTER 7

Prevention Strategies

H. Pylori Eradication

Eliminating Helicobacter pylori (H. pylori) from the digestive tract is one of the most important methods for avoiding peptic ulcers. H. Because it weakens the stomach and duodenum's protective lining and increases their vulnerability to injury from stomach acid, H. pylori is a significant cause of peptic ulcers. Eliminating this bacteria drastically lowers the chance of ulcer development and associated problems.

Usually, a combination of antibiotics and drugs that lower acid is used in the eradication procedure. Typically, doctors will give antibiotics like metronidazole, clarithromycin, and amoxicillin to eradicate the H. pylori microbes.

Proton pump inhibitors (PPIs) and H2-receptor antagonists, which lessen the production of stomach acid and foster an environment that is less favorable to bacterial development, are often administered in conjunction with antibiotics.

To guarantee that H is completely eradicated, it is essential to take antibiotics as directed by a medical professional for the whole specified duration. pylori. Antibiotic resistance and treatment failure might result from not adhering to the prescribed course of action or from missing doses. Furthermore, if the first course of therapy fails because of antibiotic resistance, some patients could need other combinations of antibiotics.

Ensuring the effective elimination of H and monitoring its efficacy during therapy requires regular follow-up visits with healthcare specialists. pylori. To verify bacterial clearance, follow-up testing, such as breathalyzers or stool antigen tests, can be carried out. Should H. pylori survive the first treatment, several rounds of antibiotics could be required to completely eradicate the infection and stop ulcer recurrence.

Reducing The Use Of Nsaids

In addition to being often used to treat pain and inflammation, nonsteroidal anti-inflammatory medications (NSAIDs) significantly raise the risk of peptic ulcers. NSAIDs function by blocking the cyclooxygenase (COX) enzyme, which is necessary for the synthesis of prostaglandins, which help shield the stomach lining from acid erosion.

NSAIDs that suppress COX also decrease prostaglandin synthesis, which increases the stomach's susceptibility to acid reflux disease. The development of erosive gastritis, peptic ulcers, and even gastrointestinal bleeding may result from long-term or excessive usage of NSAIDs.

Limiting the use of NSAIDs is crucial to preventing ulcers caused by these drugs, particularly in high-risk persons such as elderly adults, those with a history of stomach bleeding or ulcers, and people taking many drugs that may raise the risk of ulcers.

Those who want pain treatment but run the risk of developing ulcers may benefit from other pain management techniques like acetaminophen or topical NSAIDs. Additionally, minimizing the risk of ulcer formation may be achieved by taking NSAIDs for the shortest amount of time at the lowest therapeutic dosage.

Gastroprotective drugs, such as prostaglandin analogs or PPIs, may be recommended to patients who need long-term NSAID treatment for chronic illnesses like arthritis to assist preserve the stomach lining and lower the risk of ulcer development. To reduce the risk of ulcers and associated consequences, it is crucial to carefully consider the advantages and disadvantages of NSAID medication and go through choices with a healthcare professional.

Healthy Diet And Lifestyle Habits

Preventing peptic ulcers and preserving general gastrointestinal health require adhering to a nutritious diet and lifestyle. It is essential to adopt behaviors that support stomach and digestive health since certain dietary and lifestyle variables have the potential to either enhance or lower the risk of ulcer formation.

A diet high in fruits, vegetables, healthy grains, and lean meats may support good digestion and assist provide vital nutrients. Particularly foods high in fiber may aid in controlling bowel motions and preventing constipation, both of which can hasten the formation of ulcers.

Eat less or stay away from spicy, acidic, and fatty meals since these may irritate the stomach lining and exacerbate symptoms of ulcers. Additionally, because they may aggravate the digestive system and raise the formation of stomach acid, alcohol, and caffeine should also be taken in moderation.

Apart from dietary considerations, sustaining a healthy lifestyle may also be very important in preventing ulcers. Frequent exercise has many advantages for digestive health, including better circulation, lowered stress levels, and general well-being.

The incidence of stress-induced ulcers may be decreased by practicing relaxation methods like yoga, deep breathing exercises, or meditation. Prolonged stress may impair immunity and heighten vulnerability to H. pylori infection, which makes stress reduction a crucial component in preventing ulcers.

Regular Screening For High-Risk Individuals

For those who are more susceptible to ulcers, such as those who have a history of ulcers, it is important to undergo routine screening for peptic ulcer disease. Stomach pylori infection or long-term NSAID usage. Screening early may help discover ulcers before they worsen into more serious problems and enhance the effectiveness of therapy.

Endoscopic exams, such as esophagogastroduodenoscopy (EGD) or upper gastrointestinal endoscopy, may be used as screening tools because they enable medical professionals to see within the stomach and duodenum and see any ulcers or inflammation. To check for H, biopsy samples may also be obtained during endoscopy. pylori infection or rule out any further medical issues.

Non-invasive procedures like breathalyzers and stool antigen testing may be used in addition to endoscopic screening to identify H. pylori infection in those who have a history of ulcers or who are asymptomatic. These are easy, secure, and reliable ways to diagnose H. pylori and direct the choice of therapy.

As part of their preventative healthcare practice, those who are at high risk of getting ulcers should have screenings regularly. This is because early identification and management may help avoid complications and improve long-term results. Medical professionals can evaluate a patient's risk variables and suggest suitable screening intervals in light of the patient's medical history and risk profile.

CHAPTER 8

Diet And Nutrition

Foods To Avoid (Spicy, Acidic)

Knowing which foods to avoid to prevent symptoms from becoming worse is essential for controlling peptic ulcers. Spicy foods, however often cherished for their taste, may seriously damage stomachs prone to ulcers. Compounds included in ingredients like curry powders, spicy sauces, and chili peppers might irritate the stomach lining, perhaps increasing pain and inflammation.

In the same way, you should proceed cautiously while eating acidic meals. Acidity is high in tomatoes and tomato-based products (such as tomato sauce) and citrus fruits (such as oranges, lemons, and grapefruits). Eating these foods might increase the stomach's production of acid, which can exacerbate ulcer symptoms and delay their recovery. Due to its acidic nature, vinegar—which is often used in salad dressings and pickled foods—can also be harmful to those who have peptic ulcers.

Even while eliminating these meals can seem difficult, it's important to put your health first and choose other, ulcer-friendly choices. Thankfully, there are many delectable and healthful substitutes out now to accommodate different tastes and preferences.

Foods To Consume (Fiber-Rich, Probiotics)

On the other hand, foods that support healthy digestion and relieve the lining of the stomach may play a major role in helping to manage peptic ulcers. Rich meals that are high in fiber are important actors in this respect. Good sources of dietary fiber include fruits and vegetables like apples, berries, broccoli, and spinach, as well as whole grains like quinoa, brown rice, and oats. For those who have peptic ulcers, fiber may be very helpful as it helps control bowel motions, avoids constipation, and enhances overall digestive well-being.

Additionally, eating a diet high in foods rich in probiotics might help maintain a better environment in your stomach. When taken in sufficient quantities, living bacteria known as probiotics provide several health advantages. Probiotic-rich foods that may assist maintain gastrointestinal health and help rebalance the gut flora include yogurt, kefir, kimchi, sauerkraut, and kombucha. Probiotics have the potential to mitigate inflammation and accelerate the healing process of peptic ulcers by increasing the number of beneficial microorganisms in the digestive tract.

Meal Planning Tips For Ulcer Management

For ulcer care, creating a well-rounded diet plan is crucial to reducing symptoms and accelerating recovery. When making meal plans, keep the following useful advice in mind:

1. Balanced Plate: Make an effort to include a range of nutrient-dense foods, such as whole grains, fruits, vegetables, lean meats, and healthy fats, into each meal. This well-rounded strategy minimizes possible ulcer causes while ensuring you're reaching your nutritional requirements.

2. Small, Frequent Meals: Choose to eat smaller, more frequent meals throughout the day as opposed to big ones, which may overstress the digestive system. Eating smaller meals more often lessens the chance of pain and helps stop the formation of too much stomach acid.

3. **Mindful Eating:** Chew your meal slowly and deeply, enjoying every taste. In addition to helping with digestion, eating slowly and carefully enables you to pay attention to your body's signals of hunger and fullness, which helps you avoid overindulging and discomfort.

4. **Reduce Food Triggers:** Determine which foods make your ulcer symptoms worse and steer clear of them. Although each person has different triggers, spicy, acidic, and highly processed meals, as well as alcohol and caffeine, are often identified causes.

5. **Keep Yourself Hydrated:** Sustaining good digestive and general health requires being well hydrated. Drink as much water as possible throughout the day, and think about including hydrating items in your meals and snacks, such as fruits and vegetables.

You may improve the way you manage your peptic ulcers and maintain your general health by implementing these meal planning recommendations into your everyday routine.

Hydration Importance

It is very important to stay hydrated, particularly for those who are taking care of peptic ulcers. Sustaining mucosal integrity, promoting proper digestive function, and speeding up the healing of stomach ulcers all depend on adequate hydration.

Water is essential for several physiological functions in the body, such as nutrition absorption and digestion. Water consumption facilitates the easy passage of food through the digestive system, reducing the risk of constipation and encouraging regular bowel movements. This is especially important for those who have peptic ulcers since constipation may make symptoms worse and slow down the healing process.

Additionally, drinking plenty of water supports the integrity of the stomach's protective layer, the gastric mucosa. The likelihood of ulcer development and aggravation is decreased when the mucosal barrier is well-hydrated since it is more resilient to the corrosive effects of stomach acid and other irritants.

Apart from just plain water, foods high in water content, such as fruits and vegetables, may help you meet your daily fluid needs and also provide vital vitamins, minerals, and antioxidants. Adding items high in water content, such as spinach, cucumbers, melons, and strawberries, to your diet will enhance your attempts to stay hydrated and promote general health.

To sum up, keeping your stomach healthy and treating peptic ulcers both depend on drinking enough water. Through the use of water and meals high in moisture, people may help promote the healing process, reduce symptoms, and preserve excellent digestive health.

CHAPTER 9

Coping And Support

Psychological Impact Of Peptic Ulcers

Peptic ulcers may hurt a person's mental health in addition to their physical symptoms. Anxiety, despair, and frustration may result from having to cope with continual pain, suffering, and lifestyle changes. Imagine going to bed every day not knowing whether you'll be able to eat without experiencing excruciating agony or suffering afterwards. This uncertainty may lead to a heavy psychological cost.

Stress levels might also increase due to the worry of consequences like bleeding or perforation. Peptic ulcer sufferers often struggle to sleep at night or focus because of anxiety related to their illness. The effects could not stop with the ulcerated person; they might also affect others close to them, making them feel worried or powerless about their well-being.

Healthcare professionals and caregivers must comprehend the psychosocial effects of peptic ulcers. Acknowledging the emotional difficulties linked to the illness, they may provide suitable assistance and measures to enhance the patient's general welfare.

Stress Management Techniques

Since stress is known to make peptic ulcer symptoms worse, addressing the illness requires adopting efficient stress management skills. People may use a variety of techniques to lower their stress levels and encourage relaxation.

Exercises involving deep breathing are one method that is often advised. People may assist reduce stress and tension by concentrating on taking calm, deep breaths, which triggers the body's relaxation response. Additional useful techniques for relaxing the mind and lowering stress levels include mindfulness exercises and meditation.

Regular physical exercise may also help lower stress and enhance general well-being. Examples of this include swimming, yoga, and walking. Exercise improves sleep quality and produces endorphins, which are naturally occurring mood enhancers. These benefits are particularly helpful in the treatment of peptic ulcers.

It's also critical for people to recognize and deal with the causes of stress in their lives. Discovering effective coping mechanisms for stresses, such as work-related pressure, marital problems, or financial concerns, might help stop them from escalating symptoms of peptic ulcers.

Communicating With Healthcare Providers

To effectively manage peptic ulcers and provide the best possible treatment, effective communication with healthcare professionals is crucial. It should be easy for patients to talk to their healthcare team about their symptoms, worries, and preferred course of treatment.

It's critical to be upfront and truthful about symptoms and how they affect day-to-day functioning when speaking with medical professionals. Maintaining a symptom journal may be useful for identifying trends and giving medical professionals precise information when necessary.

Additionally, patients need to feel free to clarify any doubts they may have regarding their illness and course of therapy by asking questions. Patients may make more educated decisions regarding their care if they are aware of the possible side effects and the reasoning behind treatment choices.

Patients may use other tools to be informed and involved in their treatment in addition to verbal communication. This might include reading information from trustworthy sources, such as respectable websites or instructional materials supplied by medical professionals.

People with peptic ulcers may get individualized treatment that takes into account their particular requirements and preferences by encouraging open communication and cooperation between patients and healthcare professionals. To improve quality of life and get the greatest potential results, this relationship is necessary.

CHAPTER 10

Living With Peptic Ulcers

Long-Term Outlook

Managing the illness well and being aware of the long-term prognosis are important aspects of living with peptic ulcers. Although peptic ulcers may be managed and symptoms reduced, if appropriate measures aren't followed, they could return. To guarantee a bright future, it is essential to take a proactive stance.

Following a successful course of therapy, patients should schedule routine follow-up visits with their doctor to keep an eye out for any indications of recurrence. During these consultations, medical experts may evaluate how well the therapy is working and make any required changes to avoid flare-ups in the future.

They also provide patients a chance to talk about any worries or changes in their symptoms.

When it comes to modifying their lifestyle, people with peptic ulcers should concentrate on eating a balanced diet, controlling their stress levels, and avoiding situations that can make their symptoms worse. This might include giving up drinking, quitting smoking, and, if at all possible, staying away from nonsteroidal anti-inflammatory medicines (NSAIDs).

Additionally, managing stress levels may help prevent ulcer formation or recurrence. Stress-relieving practices like yoga, meditation, or regular exercise might assist achieve this. To promote long-term ulcer treatment, self-care, and general well-being must be given priority.

People may greatly enhance their long-term prognosis and lower their chance of recurrence by controlling their peptic ulcers with diligence and proactivity. Many individuals with peptic ulcers may live healthy, fulfilling lives free from recurrent flare-ups with the correct lifestyle changes and continued medical treatment.

Monitoring For Recurrence

One of the most important parts of having peptic ulcers is keeping an eye out for recurrence. If appropriate measures aren't implemented, ulcers may recur even after effective treatment. As a result, people should continue to be watchful and aware of any changes in their pain or symptoms.

Scheduling regular follow-up meetings with medical professionals is crucial for keeping an eye on the disease and identifying any early warning signals of recurrence. To examine the stomach lining and spot any ulcer development, medical personnel may use diagnostic procedures like endoscopy or imaging scans during these visits.

To assist detect possible triggers or warning indications of ulcer recurrence, people may follow their symptoms and dietary habits at home in addition to receiving medical care. Keeping a meal journal and recording any episodes of bloating, indigestion, or stomach discomfort might reveal important trends and causes.

Furthermore, to reduce the chance of an ulcer recurring, it's essential to follow the recommended course of action and dosage. Taking H2-receptor antagonists or proton pump inhibitors (PPIs) as directed by medical professionals may fall under this category.

People who are proactive and mindful of their health may successfully track the recurrence of ulcers and take the necessary precautions to avoid flare-ups. To manage peptic ulcers and preserve a high standard of living, early identification and management are essential.

Quality Of Life Considerations

Peptic ulcers may affect a person's nutrition, social life, and general well-being, among other elements of everyday living. As such, quality of life considerations must be taken into account while managing the disease and modifying lifestyle choices.

Dietary changes are an important part of helping people with peptic ulcers live better lives. While certain meals and drinks might aggravate ulcer symptoms or cause new ones, others can ease pain and encourage recovery. Collaborating with medical professionals or dietitians is crucial in creating a customized eating regimen that satisfies dietary requirements and reduces symptoms associated with ulcers.

For those who have peptic ulcers, self-care practices, and stress management may greatly enhance quality of life in addition to dietary modifications. Stress may make ulcer symptoms worse and has been related to increased stomach acid output. Thus, adding stress-relieving practices like mindfulness, deep breathing, or hobbies may aid in lowering stress and enhancing general well-being.

Having a strong support system of friends, family, and medical experts may also be very helpful in providing emotional support and motivation when managing an ulcer. Using support groups or online forums to connect with others who have gone through similar things may help foster understanding and a feeling of kinship.

Overall, the key to enhancing quality of life while dealing with peptic ulcers is to prioritize self-care, manage stress, and ask for help from loved ones and medical experts. People may improve their health and more effectively manage their illness by taking proactive measures to address these variables.

Resources For Ongoing Education And Support

For those who have peptic ulcers, it is essential to have access to services for continuing education and support. Throughout the ulcer treatment process, these sites may provide insightful advice, emotional support, and helpful information.

Patient education resources from respected medical organizations or healthcare practitioners are a great resource for people with peptic ulcers. Brochures, websites, and educational films covering a range of ulcer treatment topics, such as food suggestions, prescription details, and lifestyle advice, may be among these resources.

Furthermore, people with peptic ulcers may find a feeling of belonging and community in support groups or online discussion boards. People may ask questions, assist one another, and share their experiences on these channels. Talking to others who are aware of the difficulties associated with having an ulcer may be powerful and comforting.

In addition, medical professionals are essential in offering peptic ulcer sufferers continuing education and assistance. It should be easy for patients to communicate their worries, ask questions, and seek advice from their medical team. For ulcer therapy to be successful, patients and physicians must collaborate and communicate openly.

Finally, keeping up with the most recent findings and advancements in ulcer management and therapy may enable people to make knowledgeable choices regarding their care. This may include reading and keeping up with medical publications, going to conferences or seminars, or following reliable websites for news and updates on medicine.

Through the use of many resources for continuous education and assistance, people suffering from peptic ulcers may improve their understanding, proficiency, and self-assurance in efficiently managing their illness. A thorough support network, ranging from patient education materials to support groups and medical professionals, may significantly impact the ulcer treatment process.

CONCLUSION

To sum up, peptic ulcers are a common gastrointestinal ailment marked by erosions in the stomach or upper section of the small intestine. Numerous causes, including Helicobacter pylori infection, overuse of nonsteroidal anti-inflammatory medications (NSAIDs), smoking, and stress, may cause these ulcers.

Over time, improvements in medical knowledge and care have changed how peptic ulcers are managed. We now know that H plays a key part in this, contrary to previous theories that suggested stress and spicy meals were the main causes. NSAID usage with H. pylori infection. A patient's medical history, physical examination, and diagnostic procedures like endoscopy, biopsy, or imaging investigations are usually used in conjunction with one another to make a diagnosis.

The goals of treatment plans for peptic ulcers are to eliminate H, reduce symptoms, encourage ulcer healing, and avoid complications. pylori infection, should it exist. The cornerstones of treatment include proton pump inhibitors (PPIs), H2 receptor antagonists, antibiotics, and lifestyle changes. Furthermore, ulcer healing and recurrence prevention may be facilitated by avoiding NSAIDs and practicing stress management.

Severe peptic ulcer complications might include bleeding, perforation, and blockage. On the other hand, prompt diagnosis and effective treatment greatly lower the chance of problems and enhance patient outcomes.

In addition, it is critical to educate patients about the significance of medication compliance, lifestyle changes, and routine follow-up to avoid ulcer recurrence and preserve general gastrointestinal health.

Even though peptic ulcers may be difficult to cure, advances in medical understanding and available therapeutic options have significantly improved patient outcomes. Healthcare providers may successfully treat peptic ulcers and reduce the risk of complications by using a holistic strategy that includes medical therapy, lifestyle adjustments, and patient education. This will eventually improve the quality of life for those who are impacted by this ailment.

THE END

www.ingramcontent.com/pod-product-compliance
Lightning Source LLC
Chambersburg PA
CBHW070315230526
45470CB00002B/893